Life After Stroke

One Man's Journey Through Recovery

George Tsatsu Tamakloe

Publisher: George Tsatsu Tamakloe
Email: nagava01@gmail.com
Photos Credits: Osscar Diaz & Tamara Griebell
Front Cover Photo & Bio Headshot: Tamara Griebell

I DEDICATE THIS BOOK
TO THE FOLLOWING PEOPLE

MARK EFUI TAMAKLOE

ALBERTA ABLAH ABUI TAMAKLOE

AGBEKO TSIKATA (AKA CARLOS)

JOHN BENJAMIN ANNOH-QUARSHIE

CHOCHO LASSEY

SEFAKOR AFI MENSAH

VERONICA ADJETEY

TABLE OF CONTENTS

ACKNOWLEDGMENTS

I would like to acknowledge my amazing children

MARK TAMAKLOE

ARLYTHEA TAMAKLOE

DEEP APPRECIATION TO THE
PEOPLE WHO HAVE BEEN BY MY SIDE SINCE
MY STROKE

BRIGID KOKUI TAMAKLOE

RASHID RAJI

PAPA FREE INTERNET

JACKIE RAJI

PHLIP ACOLATSE

EYRAM TAMAKLOE

SOLOMON WAB-LUMOR

EDDIE ANANE-AKOLLOR

JONES ATSRIKU-AGYEMAN

BOTCHWAY NORTEI

DEGANUS TEO

DOGBATSE DEVINE

FOKUO KWAME

GEORGE KORLEY (CASANOVA)

LARRY MENSAH

ROSEMARY MENSAH

PAUL NYARKO

GEORGE OFORI-AMANFO (Zibello)
FRANCIS OHEMEN-ADU
SAMUEL OKOE
SAM WADEE
JACOB ZWENNES
PETER ZWENNES
ZACH ABRAHAM
VERA ADDY
KWAME FOXUE
NORTEY BOTCHWAY
ERNEST TANSON
HYDER QUARSHIE
AUDREY QUAYE
HYDER TRABOULSI
SYLVIA DAGANUS
OKO TITUS-GLOVER
TONY ADEDZE
EDEM TSIKATA
GEORGE GYAN
GEORGE COFIE
TINA SENIOR
STEVENS AMPATEY
CHARLES ODEI
FRANCIS ALLAH BOAKYE
DANIEL AKAKPO
AURELIA AKAKPO
SELASI AKAKPO
ELIZABETH ACOLATSE
KENNY

YMCA FRIENDS

DENISE BUCCIERO
JERRICA KULBIS
BRIDGID ROTHENBERG
BRENDA WERNEIWSKEI
LISA MCGOVERN
KENNETH CARDULLO
TIA HOPKINS
CAROL PERROTTA
CHUCK LAMBERY
TAMARA GRIEBELL
OSCAR DIAZ
LORNA RIFKIN
ELENA THOMAS
TRACY SALVESEN
ANNE DEGENNARO
CHRIS WADHERA
DEMME MATHEOS
JOHN ABAIR
KRISTIN DUFNER

INTRODUCTION

Looking forward to another day in the office, George Tsatsu Tamakloe retired to bed.

Earlier that evening he had been going through his usual paces, addressing his workload for the following morning. Little did he know that he would be leaving his office that evening for the very last time. Tsatsu, as he is called by his friends and family, woke up the following day in a hospital bed.

After he regained consciousness, he was told that he had suffered a stroke during the night. This turn of events altered the trajectory of his life for good.

George still loves and enjoys life to the fullest even though he had to learn how to walk, talk, read, and write all over again. As he slowly recovered in the intensive care unit, his friends and family immediately recognized how important it would be for George to get rehabilitation therapy as soon as possible.

This would increase his chances of a recovery that allowed him to regain his independence which was one of the things he asked God to provide. At this point it was very clear there was a direct correlation between the speed of recovery, rehabilitation, and the cost of treatment.

Ten years down the road, Tsatsu has partially regained his independence and is very appreciative of the support his friends gave him on his long road to recovery. This book is his way of expressing his gratitude to friends and family who have stayed by his side and supported his search for independence and happiness.

CHAPTER 1
Live the Best Life

I met Rashid Raji in Ghana when I was a teenager. He was in his twenties at the time. When I would walk to the bus to go to school, I would see him sitting outside of the tailor shop. It was the place where young people would hang out. I would chat with him before catching my bus. He had moved to America to attend college. Once he graduated he started a business in Ghana and traveled back and forth.

I moved to America when I was 20 years old. I lived with my brother in Chicago and then I moved to New York where I worked and attended college for 3 years. Rashid and I had stayed in touch so when I moved to New Jersey we started hanging out together.

We have been friends for 30 some years. Whenever I need help, Rashid is there. As soon as he found out about my stroke, he headed for the hospital. He visited me every day. Once I got home, he would stop by my house before he went to work.

Five years after my stroke, Rashid moved into his home in North Carolina. Even though he had his house in New Jersey up for sale, he took it off the market and allowed me to stay there for 5 years. This was after my stroke as I was going through my divorce. When I was financially able to move into a condo, he put his house up for sale.

Rashid set up what I needed medically, made phone calls for me, and set up the transportation that I needed in order to go to the YMCA three days a week.

I used to work in accounting and finance so I would help Rashid in those areas. My ability to help him has decreased, however I still help him in any way I can. We are more than friends, we are brothers.

I would imagine that you know someone who has been the victim of a stroke.

Strokes are a major health problem. For example in England, over 200,000 people have a stroke every year and it is the third largest cause of death, after heart diseases and cancer.

The brain damage caused by strokes means that strokes are the largest cause of adult disability. In fact, stroke occurs every 10 minutes and can instantly change lives at any time and at any age.

In August 2008, a stroke nearly took my life and it changed my whole world. I was rushed to the hospital for immediate medical attention after collapsing in my bathroom.

I am thankful for the good medical care I received in the US and the love and support from my family and friends in the United States, United Kingdom, and Ghana. I am also thankful to God that I am still alive.

I am living proof that you can survive a stroke and that rehabilitation is not a waste of time. No matter what disabilities you have, you can still contribute.

My mobility and motor skills have greatly improved as a result of joining the gym, improving my diet, and widening my social circles.

While in hospital I had a second stroke and it affected my brain. I have issues with my short term memory and I was diagnosed with aphasia.

The following information is from the American Speech-Language-Hearing Association (ASHA).

Aphasia

- Difficulty speaking
- Trouble understanding speech
- Difficulty with word recall
- Problems with reading or writing

CHAPTER 2
Do the Best You Can

Don't give up on life. I remember one thing that my grandmother taught me: As you are going up in life, never forget the people who are below you because you will meet them again as you are coming down, should you fall. If you are not nice to them, they will not help you when you're down.

When I had my stroke, many people came to see me and they always asked how they could help me.

Friends contributed to buy me a comfortable chair and many other things.
- Visited me and helped me with anything I needed at the time
- Drove me places

The Catholic Church was also very helpful and supportive.
- Delivered canned food to me
- Provided rides to church when needed

The YMCA played a huge part in my recovery. I help out there because I believe in giving back. This facility became my second home. The members and staff became my second family.

Swimming

I never knew how to swim until I started my recovery process at the YMCA.

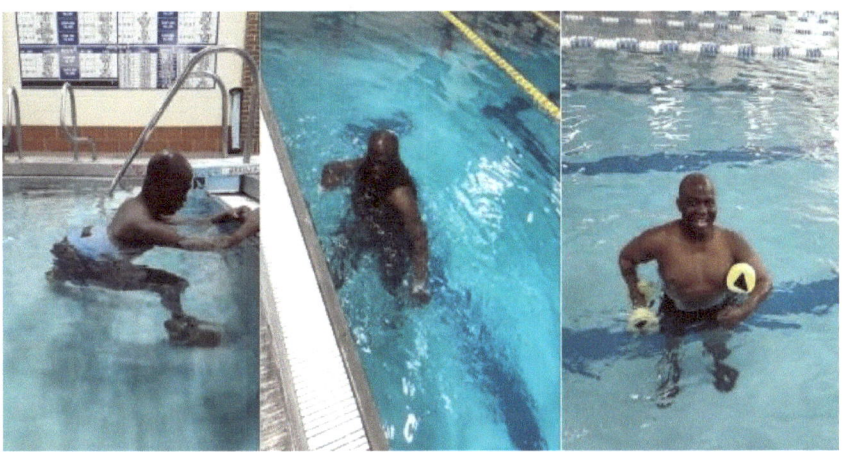

Boxing

Some days I do boxing and other days I train on the treadmill or with other muscle strengthening equipment.

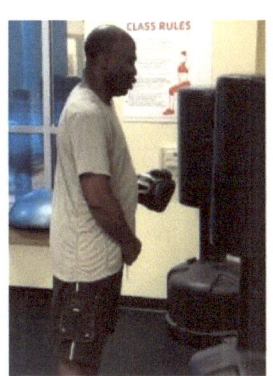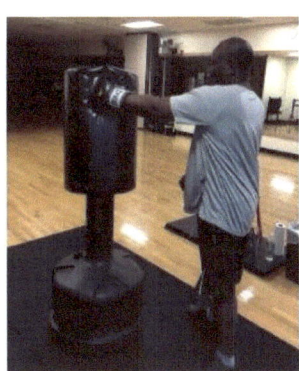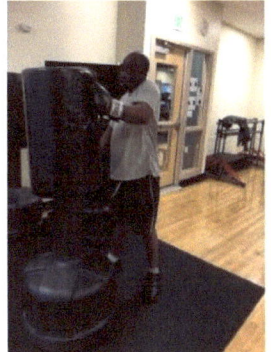

Other Exercises I Do At The YMCA

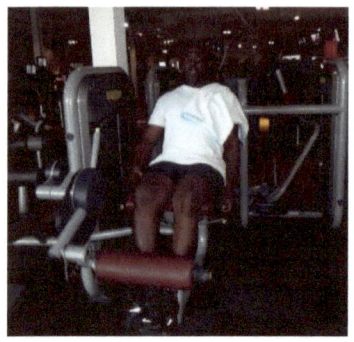
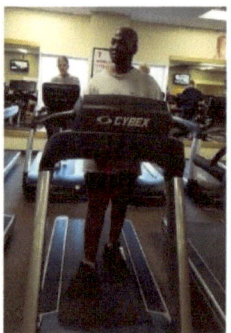
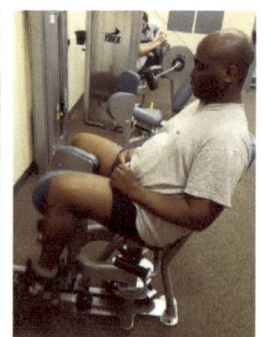

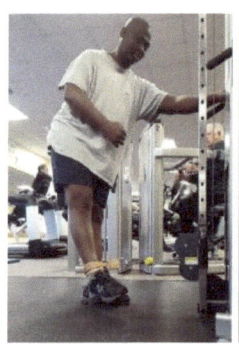
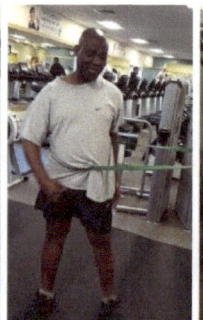
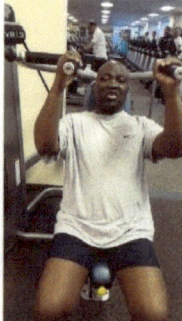
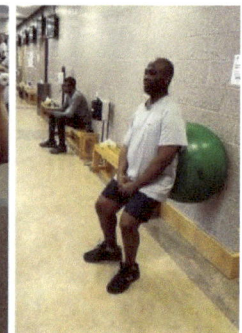

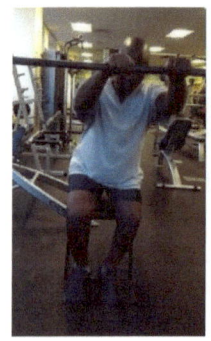
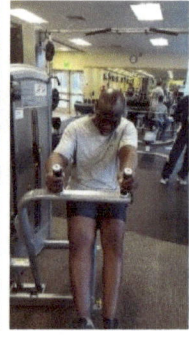
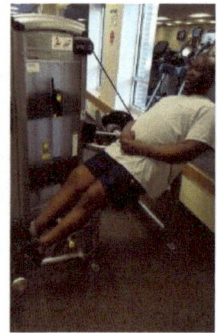
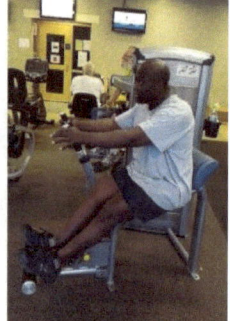

Relaxing In The Whirlpool

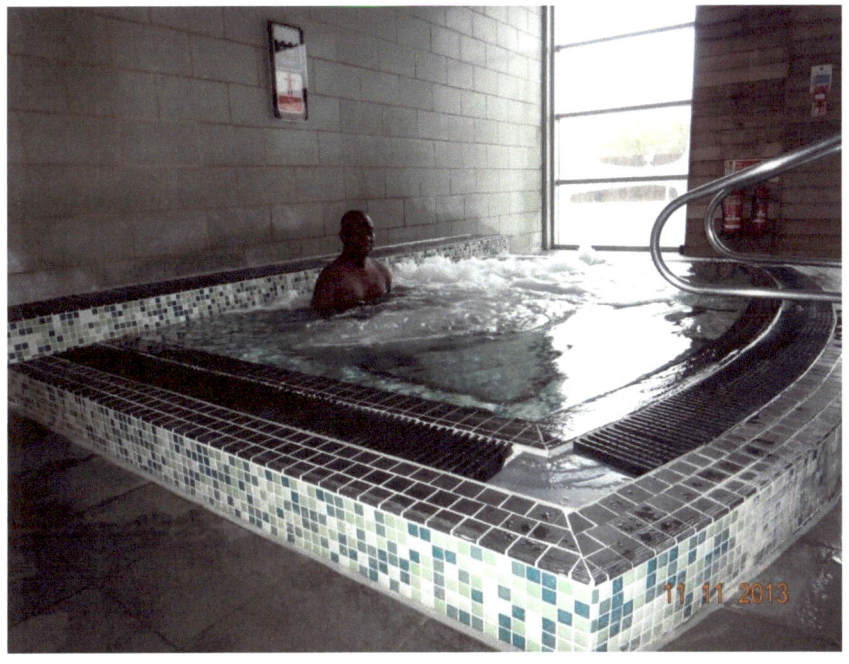

CHAPTER 3
Help People Around You

When I was in high school I recall helping anyone I could. I grew up being told to be kind to people. There are many ways to help others.

In Ghana I was given a scholarship to attend school. I met some really great guys there: Francis, Peter, Zibello, Jacob, and other friends.

When I moved to America and was working, my attitude was that no work is below me. I also made sure to send money back home in order to help out.

I worked longer hours if necessary. If I needed more training I took a class, even if it was out of my own pocket. This is how I helped myself and my boss.

I have two kids in college right now. Their schooling has been very important for me. My son's name is Mark (Efui). He attended Princeton University for his pre-med studies. Now he is finishing his Master's Degree at the University of Pennsylvania. He is planning on becoming a doctor.

My daughter's name is Arlythea. She is attending a fashion school in Manhattan, New York.

I coached both of them in soccer. They also enjoyed tennis, karate, and basketball. They know how to swim, which is something I wish I had learned myself before my stroke.

Even though their mom and I are no longer together, I don't hold any grudges against her. I keep things peaceful for the sake of my kids.

In our marriage we took turns. I dropped the kids off at school on my way to work and my wife picked them up.

I used to cook because my father's sister taught me and I enjoy cooking.

I helped with the laundry and made sure I washed my own clothes, eventually I taught my kids to wash their own clothes.

On Saturdays, I would help clean the house and mow the lawn. Weekends were also the time for driving my kid's to sports games.

I taught my kids that if you tell someone you are going to help them, make sure you follow through.

Family is very important to me. That is another place where we can help others. My mother-in-law came to visit and help out, just before my first child was born. Six months later she took him back to Ghana with her. My mother brought him back six months later. She stayed with us for one year. When it was time for her to leave, my wife and I put our son in daycare. When my daughter was born my wife stayed home with her for the first four months of her life. Then we put her in daycare as well to join her brother.

CHAPTER 4
Enjoy Life

I love to travel. Family trips were always very special for me. We went to California to see Disneyland and to Florida to tour Disney World.

Everyone enjoyed traveling to the Bahamas.

I love to listen to Jazz on my laptop, a CD or the radio.

I like all kinds of music including Blues, Western, Jamaican (Bob Marley), Hispanic, French, African, and Classical.

I love to learn...

Early School
I was born in Ghana, Africa. When I was 4 years old I went to live with my grandmother in Lomé, Togo, Africa. My mother and father stayed in Ghana for work. After attending primary school in Togo, I moved back to Ghana to continue with middle school education. I had forgotten how to speak English, Ga, and Ewe, the languages I spoke when I was 4 years old and living in Ghana. So I brought with me a

language barrier when I moved back to Ghana at age 11. I only spoke a Togolese dialect and French. Everywhere I went, including school and even at playgrounds, I had to depend on others to translate for me.

I spent one year in Primary School and passed the test.

I continued to St. Aquinas Secondary School in Accra for five years. Didn't do well on the final O'level exams and had to retake the exams the following year which I passed with distinction. I met my good friend Nii Adamafio at Accra Academy Secondary School where I studied to retake the O'level exams.

I was accepted at St. Augustine Secondary School, in Cape Coast, Africa where I completed my post high school sixth form...

College

-Attended 3 years of college at the prestigious Kwame Nkrumah University of Science and Technology (KNUST) in Kumasi, Ghana

-Had the opportunity to come to America and teach people about Africa. I stayed with my cousin in Chicago, Illinois for 6 months. Finished the last year of college when I moved to New York (Baruch

College) and went on to get a Master's Degree at Long Island University

-Drove for Yellow Cab in New York City to support myself and ran errands for a firm in NYC

-First Job after graduation, company got sold and I was let go

-Second Job worked for a company in NJ

After College
-Extra classes for work and Community Education

Resume

I have included my resume on the following 3 pages so that you can see I was able to do many things before my stroke.

GEORGE T. TAMAKLOE

BUSINESS SYSTEMS ANALYST ~ FINANCIAL SYSTEMS ANALYST

Cost/Benefits Analysis...Variance Analysis & Projection... Investment Analysis
Project Management... Financial Planning & Budgeting...Taxation
Securities Markets...Investment Instruments... Product Development

Remarkable track record leveraging technology expertise to improve process, accuracy, return-time and cost retention within large-scale business and financial systems. Dynamic understanding of system integrations, upgrades, deployment, implementation and applications development. Outstanding team-building, leadership, and communications skills utilized in delivering countless presentations and meetings, and collaborating with business and technology counterparts during client project analysis and problem resolution. Superior knowledge of various investment instruments, including equities, fixed income securities, Repos, Swaps, Options, Derivatives, Asset – Backed and Mortgage-Backed Securities, Hedge Funds and Mutual Funds; and Trading Systems such as Charles River, McGregor, Bloomberg, Merrin, Global One, and SunGard.

TECHNICAL APPLICATIONS

Languages: C Language, Visual Basic, ASP, HTML, XML, Java and JDBC.

Software: Rational Rose, Rational Unified Process, RequisitePro, UCM (Clear Case/Clear Quest), VISIO and ERWIN, Lotus Notes, MS-Office Suite, MS Project, and Crystal Reports.

Operating Systems: UNIX Windows (XP, NT and 2000).

Databases: Oracle, Sybase, IBM DB2.

Additional Knowledge: JD Edwards, Solomon and Computron with Report Writer, IBM Content Management OnDemand, McCormack & Dodge (now GEAC), business analysis, project management, financial systems conversion and implementation, systems analysis, database designs, workflow, systems testing, UML and Data modeling, Multi-Currency Accounting System (MARS), Sungard Trading and Asset management System, Portfolio Accounting System (DST), ePAM Accounting System, HedgeTek Partnership Allocation System, Bloomberg and Charles River Investment Management System.

PROFESSIONAL EXPERIENCE

Senior Business Analyst (Global Application Development Group)   07/2007 to Present
COHEN & STEERS CAPITAL MANAGEMENT INC, New York, NY

Interfaced between the Development team and the following Business Units: (Portfolio Managers, the Trading Group, Investment Administrators, the Settlement Unit and the Compliance Group). Worked with the Business Units to analyze current workflows and develop new workflows as part of the upgrade of the Charles River Investment Management System (Manager Workbench, Trading Blotter, Compliance and System Administration)

- Project Manager/Business Analyst on the initiative to upgrade the Charles River Investment Management System.
- Provided Application Support to the various Business Units, this includes the Traders, the Portfolio managers, the Settlement Group, the Investment Administrators, the Compliance Group and the Performance Group.
- Documented the current and proposed workflows for the Trading Group, Portfolio Managers, Compliance, Investment Administrators and the Settlement Unit, for the upgrade of the Charles River System.
- Prepared and performed Test cases / Scenarios for the implementation of the new version of the Charles River Investment Management System
- Interfaced with outside Vendors and Brokers to add Alternative Trading venues such as FIX Protocol, LIQUIDNET and Algorithmic Trading to the Charles River Investment Management System.

Business Analyst III, (Global Technology Service)   01/2004 to 07/2007
STATE STREET CORPORATION (Mutual Fund Services), Princeton, NJ

Effectively monitored and analyzed areas for technological improvement in the Mutual Fund Account Services and researched the available improvement sources. Additionally worked with various business units to find ways to accelerate the Merrill Lynch Investment Managements Real Time Trades Processing within its trade management system. Developed business and functional requirements for several systems to reflect SEC regulatory policies.

Continued...

Managed and coordinated various projects and technology-based solutions to meet State Street Corporation's Standards. Created test cases and validated test results during systems and user acceptance testing to ensure vision document compliance.

PROFESSIONAL EXPERIENCE ~ continued

- Researched, developed and implemented IBM's Rational Unified Process (RUP), which improved Trade Management, Portfolio Management, Pricing, General Ledger, Partnership Allocation, Shareholder Reporting and Report Distribution systems, along with Securities Processing and the Securities Holdings Database.
- Designed complex web reports portal for various applications as well as a security matrix for user entitlements.
- Successfully lobbied senior business managers in several process improvement initiatives and new product developments.
- Participated in audit reviews and execution of corrective action plans to minimize risk.

Business Analyst/AVP, Global Securities Service/RSG Technology Group   02/2001 to 01/2004
DEUTSCHE BANK (Formerly Bankers Trust), Jersey City, NJ

Functioned as liaison between the Trust accounting and Custody business lines and the Technical team during reengineering of the systems development process. Provided support by developing stored procedures for several financial instruments. Compiled and analyzed revision options for the Financial Accounting and Global Custody/Asset Management systems. Monitored the process of accounts traveling through the accounting system ensuring accuracy, timeliness, and completeness. Developed test plans for a variety of software releases. Tracked ongoing operations using key metrics and vital statistics as reference tools concentrating on quality, budget and code changes.

- Generated operating standards utilized to track and gage the new Sungard Global Plus Trading and Accounting system performance.
- Defined functional controls to monitor equities, mutual funds, fixed income, derivatives and FX contracts for a multicurrency ledger based portfolio accounting and reporting system.

Independent Consultant/Business Analyst   1999 to 2001
ERIC ROBERT AND ASSOCIATES, Deutsche Bank Account, NY
PAINE WEBBER GROUP, INC. Weehawken, NJ
LOGICAL DESIGN SOLUTIONS, New York, NY
MODIS PROFESSIONAL SERVICES, INC. (JP MORGAN & CO ACCOUNT), New York, NY

Acted as consultant for several projects conducting systems analysis and design, project management, financial analysis, writing business specifications and requirements, and product development.

- Developed business rules and key statutory requirements that influence global financial products.
- Performed analysis in the development of investment banking and financial planning internet applications.

Associate/Business Analyst (Bell Atlantic Mobile Account)   1998 to 1999
ELECTRONIC DATA SYSTEMS, BEDMINSTER, NJ

Assisted management in tracking financial developments for various projects, technical and business support for a three-tiered billing system; and compiling monthly VISION billing project status reports. Provided additional information on the VISION system including performance, reliability, and customer utilization. Conducted cost/benefit analysis reports for clients determining business and technology requirements. Worked with senior programming team during database updating and maintenance and with disaster recovery activities improving accuracy and timeliness.

Senior Accountant   1994 to 1998
NEW YORK MERCANTILE EXCHANGE, NEW YORK, NY

Prepared consolidated financial statements in compliance with internal and external standards, financial and operating reports, and profitability and analytical market reports. Assessed the ROI of numerous securities portfolios. Created profitability / analytical market reports and associated schedules on trends for management.

- Directed month- and year-end closings, and monitored financial aspects of $220 million NYMEX relocation project.
- Designed in cooperation with the technical developers a new accounting system, increasing the control and efficiency qualities.

PROFESSIONAL EXPERIENCE ~ continued

Staff Accountant
STERLING WINTHROP, INC., NEW YORK, NY   1990 to 1994

Managed the general ledger, fixed assets database and associated schedules. Analyzed swap investments, company exposure of foreign exchange, various product line revenue and costs, and currency hedging transaction. Tracked and prepared regular operating performance reports for several levels of management.

- Assisted in the reconciliation of database information during the implementation of a new accounting system.

EDUCATION

MBA, ACCOUNTING – Long Island University, Brooklyn, NY
BBA, Finance – Baruch College (CUNY), New York, NY

Seminars & Certifications

Mastering Requirements Management with Use Cases; Brokerage Operations, Hedge Funds, Financial Statement Analysis, Asset-Backed Securities, Global Securities Service, Mortgage-Backed Securities, Securities Processing; DB2 SQL & Application Programming; Systems Analysis and Design, C Programming, UNIX, Sybase; Visual Basic, Software Development for E-Commerce, Database Analysis and Designs, Java, JDBC, Oracle Data warehousing, Oracle Database, HTML, ASP, Perl

CHAPTER 5
The Small Things Will Fix Themselves

There is no need to get angry if something doesn't happen or if something doesn't get done when you decide it is supposed to be done or happen.

If you don't have a babysitter, stay at home.

When you can't get into work. Can you work from home? Ask your boss.

"The best way to predict your future is to create it."
                                    -Abraham Lincoln

"Folks are usually about as happy as they make their minds up to be."
                                    -Abraham Lincoln

"I've learned that people will forget what you said, people will forget what you did, but people will never forget how you made them feel."
                                    -Maya Angelou

"Nothing will work unless you do."   -Maya Angelou

"If you don't like something, change it. If you can't change it, change your attitude."   -Maya Angelou

"Love recognizes no barriers. It jumps hurdles, leaps fences, penetrates walls to arrive at its destination full of hope."   -Maya Angelou

"When you learn, teach. When you get, give."
                                    -Maya Angelou

"My mission in life is not merely to survive, but to thrive; and to do so with some passion, some compassion, some humor, and some style."
                                    -Maya Angelou

"If you can't fly then run, if you can't run then walk, if you can't walk then crawl, but whatever you do you have to keep moving forward."
                                    -Martin Luther King Jr.

CHAPTER 6
Things Happen

Don't let circumstances stop you from achieving your dreams.

"I can see how it might be possible for a man to look down upon the earth and be an atheist, but I cannot conceive how a man could look up into the heavens and say there is no God."

-Abraham Lincoln

"My concern is not whether God is on our side; my greatest concern is to be on God's side, for God is always right."

-Abraham Lincoln

"Whatever you are, be a good one."

-Abraham Lincoln

"I'm a success today because I had a friend who believed in me and I didn't have the heart to let him down." -Abraham Lincoln

"Everybody can be great ... because anybody can serve. You don't have to have a college degree to serve. You don't have to make your subject and verb agree to serve. You only need a heart full of grace. A soul generated by love." -Martin Luther King Jr.

"Never succumb to the temptation of bitterness."
-Martin Luther King Jr.

"Those who are not looking for happiness are the most likely to find it, because those who are searching forget that the surest way to be happy is to seek happiness for others." -Martin Luther King Jr.

"We must accept finite disappointment, but never lose infinite hope."
-Martin Luther King Jr.

"We must build dikes of courage to hold back the flood of fear."
-Martin Luther King Jr.

CHAPTER 7
Live a Full Life

Whatever it is you can do, do it. If my attitude had been "I had a stroke so now I can't do anything, I am worthless to everyone including me" I wouldn't have made as big of a recovery.

Focus on what you love and do it. Get out as much as you can.

I like to walk along the beach.

I love to dance. I make sure to listen to music. I still can't clap my hands very well. When I could finally sit in a chair again, I starting working on the ability to tap my foot on the floor. It took a while for that ability to come back to me.

Traveling is my idea of living a full life. My next trip will be to Australia and New Zealand.

I enjoy helping others anyway I can.

I used to help my friends and family move furniture. I would also use my SUV to help them move.

I knew how to fix computers so I would be the computer tech guy for my friends and family.

I coached soccer for my kid's soccer teams.

I assisted in Bingo nights at church. I ran the tables and set up the volunteers.

I used to set up chairs for church bazaars.

Now my volunteer work involves...

Being at the YMCA 3 days a week. I make sure the bathrooms are clean and that the toilets have been flushed. I pick up the mail and I clean the toys in the nursery.

When I help out at church for Bingo night, I sell tickets.

I would like to set up a facility in Ghana for victims of stroke so they can take classes and do exercises. They will also be able to find out about volunteer opportunities in their communities.

CHAPTER 8
Exercise

While in intensive care, the nurses would move my arms and legs. About a week later, I had another stroke which affected my brain. I was diagnosed with Aphasia. I now have trouble remembering the details of what I read or directions someone has given. The second stroke affected my short-term memory.

Once I got out of intensive care, I spent 5 months in the hospital and continued to get physical, occupational, and speech therapy.

After being released from the hospital I was able to attend rehabilitative therapy for 6 months through insurance, because of the benefits from where my wife worked.

I bought a stationary bike so I could ride it for 1 hour once or twice a day. I got a little better, but I was getting bored at home. I joined the YMCA. Initially I didn't work out. I just volunteered. One of the ladies at the welcome desk mentioned that swimming might be good for me. I didn't know how to swim. My boss Chuck thought it might be a good idea to workout poolside, then attempt some therapy in the water. My biggest gains came from working out at the YMCA.

Besides swimming, I do things like boxing, walking on the treadmill, as well as weight training. Core training has been very helpful for me to regain my balance.

I am grateful to the staff and members of the Old Bridge YMCA for their help and support. The mission of the YMCA: To collaborate and work together on areas of mutual benefit in order to strengthen and enhance our individual YMCAs.

Stretching (arms and legs, standing and sitting)

Laying on my back (alternately crossing my legs)

On my stomach (arching my back with my feet up)

CHAPTER 9
Travel the World

Born in Ghana
Went to French school in Togo (returned to Ghana)

Chicago, Illinois, USA
My cousin lives in Chicago. I stayed with him when I first came to America.

Bahamas
British Island with my wife for our honeymoon. After having kids we stayed on one island and took boat trips to the other islands.

California
Disneyland as a family and then the kids stayed with a relative there and went to Disneyland many other times.

Washington DC
I took my family to Washington DC. We saw the cathedral and took a bus tour that stopped at museums and art galleries.

Virginia
We ate crabs in Virginia and took my kids to a baseball game.

Florida
NASA space station in Cape, Canaveral
Disney World
MGM Studios
Epcot Center

United Kingdom
My sister lives in Cambridge, which is in Great Britain so I stayed with her at different times on my way to visit family in Ghana.

1 year after my stroke, I stopped in London on my way to seeing my mom in Ghana.

South Africa
3 years after my stroke, I traveled from South Africa, north along the coast by bus. It was a 2 week trip.

London
When I was going through my divorce, 5 years after my stroke my nephew, my sister's, son took me to London for a bus tour.

France
I walked to the top of the Eiffel Tower. Paris is where I stopped on my way to Ghana to visit my family when I was 40 years old.

CHAPTER 10
Understand Others

I believe it is important to take the time to listen to what people have to say before making any judgment.

Once you understand their situation you can make a better judgment.

If you have anything to offer them and they are open to advice, then give it to them.

I try very hard not to be judgmental. I realize that everybody's situation is different.

Attempting to see things through another person's eyes is helpful in creating strong relationships. Seeing things from their perspective creates empathy for others.

I do my best to make friends with everyone and I don't judge people by their color or religion.

After my stroke I realized that my voice would go up to higher pitches. People understand me better when I keep my voice low and talk slowly. This works both ways.

Aphasia
Common signs and symptoms of aphasia include the following:

Impairments in Spoken Language Expression. I have difficulty finding words (Anomia)
Impairments in Spoken Language Comprehension
Impairments in Written Expression (Agraphia)
Impairments in Reading Comprehension (Alexia)

Having difficulty finding words (Anomia)

Speaking haltingly or with effort
Speaking in single words (e.g., names of objects)
Speaking in short, fragmented phrases
Omitting smaller words like the, of, and was (i.e., telegraphic speech)
Making grammatical errors
Putting words in the wrong order
Substituting sounds or words (e.g., "table" for bed; "wishdasher" for dishwasher)
Making up words (e.g., jargon)
Fluently stringing together nonsense words and real words, but leaving out or including an insufficient amount of relevant content

Impairments in Spoken Language Comprehension

Having difficulty understanding spoken utterances
Requiring extra time to understand spoken messages
Providing unreliable answers to "yes/no" questions

Failing to understand complex grammar (e.g., "The dog was chased by the cat.")

Finding it very hard to follow fast speech (e.g., radio or television news)

Misinterpreting subtleties of language (e.g., taking the literal meaning of figurative speech such as "It's raining cats and dogs.")

Lacking awareness of errors

Impairments in Written Expression (Agraphia)

Having difficulty writing or copying letters, words, and sentences

Writing single words only

Substituting incorrect letters or words

Spelling or writing nonsense syllables or words

Writing run-on sentences that don't make sense

Writing sentences with incorrect grammar

Impairments in Reading Comprehension (Alexia)

Having difficulty comprehending written material

Having difficulty recognizing some words by sight

Having the inability to sound out words

Substituting associated words for a word (e.g., "chair" for couch)

Having difficulty reading non-content words (e.g., function words such as to, from, the

Aphasia symptoms vary in severity of impairment and impact on communication, depending on factors such as the location and extent of damage and the demands of the speaking situation.

Aphasia is caused by damage to the language centers of the brain. In most people, these language centers are located in the left hemisphere, but aphasia can also occur as a result of damage to the right hemisphere; this is often referred to as crossed aphasia, to denote that the right hemisphere is language dominant in these individuals.

My aphasia is located in the right hemisphere of my brain.

Stroke is the most common cause of aphasia. According to the National Aphasia Association (n.d.), about 25%–40% of stroke survivors experience aphasia.

Speech-language pathologists (SLPs) play a central role in the screening, assessment, diagnosis, and treatment of persons with aphasia. The professional roles and activities in speech-language pathology include clinical/educational services (diagnosis, assessment, planning, and treatment); prevention and advocacy; and education, administration, and research.

ASHA is the national professional, scientific, and credentialing association for 204,000 members and affiliates who are audiologists; speech-language pathologists; speech, language, and hearing scientists; audiology and speech-language pathology support personnel; and students. Audiologists specialize in preventing and assessing hearing and balance disorders as well as providing audiologic treatment, including hearing aids. Speech-language pathologists identify, assess, and treat speech and language problems, including swallowing disorders.

VISION
Making effective communication, a human right, accessible and achievable for all.

MISSION
Empowering and supporting audiologists, speech-language pathologists, and speech, language, and hearing scientists through: Advancing science, setting standards, fostering excellence in professional practice, and advocating for members and those they serve.

••

I am here to encourage everyone. Whether you are a stroke survivor or a relative or friend of a stroke survivor, I am here to let you know that there is life after a stroke.

CHAPTER 11
All Cultures Have Something in Common

There are 50 different dialects spoken in Ghana, Africa. When I went to South Africa I met a Chinese woman who said that even though we speak different languages, we aspire to the same thing: To love and to be loved.

In the US you can be anything you want if you put your mind to it.

The attitude in Ghana is that it's important to stay positive and never give up.

In Togo, Africa, it's 'aim for the best'. You can achieve wonderful things, just put your mind towards it.

Stay in school is the focus in Nigeria, Africa.

Do the best that you can is the motto you might hear in Great Britain.

Take a nap, rest yourself, is the message we get from Spain and Mexico.

Sensual pleasure is a part of the French culture.

Being humble is the Scandinavian way. Don't think or act like you are special or better than anyone else (even if you actually are).

Australian
Respect for the freedom and dignity of the individual, freedom of religion, fair play, and compassion for those in need.

Russian
Sometimes a person has to sacrifice everything, even one's life, for the sake of the community.

South American
Latinos tend to be highly group-oriented. A strong emphasis is placed on family as the major source of one's identity and protection against the hardships of life.

There are many cultures in the world. I've just named a few.

CHAPTER 12
Others Are Suffering

You might think that your suffering is worse than other people's, however there is always someone who is worse off than you. Focus on helping that person. This will bring gratefulness into your life.

After my stroke the members of the Catholic Church brought food to me. I make sure to participate in their food drives.

Schooling
Some children in Africa are not able to attend school. There are organizations you can donate to that will buy them shoes or a bicycle or even feminine products.

Out of Work
Help those who are unemployed to develop new skills. Spread the word that you know someone who is looking for a certain job or is on a certain career path.

Homeless
We can volunteer at homeless shelters serving meals, listening and carrying on meaningful conversations, donating food and personal supplies.

Prisons

Instead of putting people in jail, how about if we help people so they are not tempted to do things that land them in jail?

ABOUT THE AUTHOR

I worked out at the gym at least 3 times a week. Late night snacks were common. I had no idea that was an unhealthy habit. Laying on the floor in my bathroom, unable to get up, was my wakeup call.

My mission is to let people know that there is life after stroke. This book is fulfilling my greatest dream to inspire others and to honor the people who have helped me along the road to recovery.

YOU CAN SEE MY PROGRESS
BY LOOKING AT MY EYES

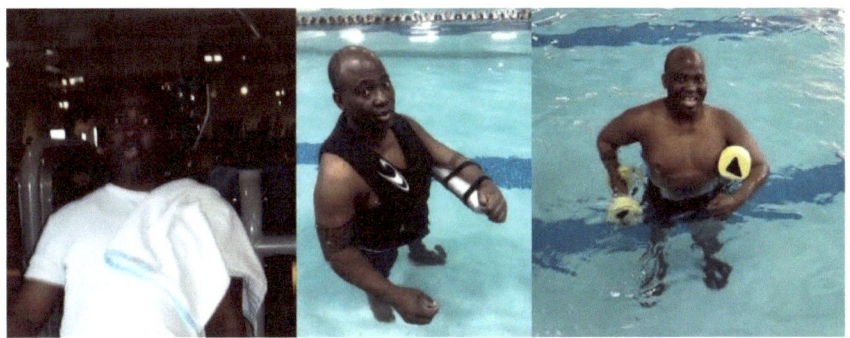

I AM LIVING PROOF THAT THERE IS LIFE AFTER STROKE

TO GOD BE THE GLORY

I sing with the song writer: To God be the glory great things he has done!

I thank God for bringing my brother George this far in the journey of life.

I give thanks to the Almighty God for the victory chalked ten years ago after falling ill with a stroke and doctors giving up on his restoration. His health is now restored and he can talk, walk, swim, and go about his life duties.

I know that the God who has brought him this far will surely perfect all that concerns him.

By Brigid Kokui Tamakloe (George's sister)

www.ingramcontent.com/pod-product-compliance
Lightning Source LLC
Chambersburg PA
CBHW041111180526
45172CB00001B/201